Knock Out Diabetes In One Month

By: Jack Kevin

Disclaimer

Reasonable care has been taken to ensure that the information presented in this book is accurate. All the information given in this book is obtained from my own research. All the information given in this book is for treating diabetes with herbal methods, however reader should understand that everything has its good and bad effects so the methods given in this book if not followed correctly will give rise to side effects
But they are not major side effects, reader should understand that if any side effect occurs then he/she will be responsible for it.

The information provided within this Book is for general informational purpose only. While we try to keep the information up-to-date and correct, there are no representations or warranties, express or implied, about the completeness, accuracy, reliability, suitability or availability with respect to the information, products, services, or related graphics contained in this Book for any purpose. Any use of this information is at your own risk.

This Book contains information that is intended to help the readers be better informed of health care. Always consult your doctor for individual needs.

The Book is not intended to be a substitute for the medical advice of licensed physician. The reader should consult with their doctor in any matters relating to his/her health.

By using anything found in this Book and using it, it is at your own risk, you take full responsibility for your actions, if you don't agree or don't want to take your own risk than is suggest you overlook this report.

Table of contents

Introduction

Hi dear readers am Jack Kevin author of "Knock Out Diabetes In One Month". Thanks appreciating my work by downloading this book

This Book provide information for treating Type I & Type II Diabetes with herbal methods and eliminating it from the body forever and it will never let them happen to form again in future. The information in this Book is

Collected from my own personal research and specially the Indian Veda called Ayurveda and all the information in this Book is told by Indian sages and you will never get this information elsewhere because the all information was in Hindi language and ancient Sanskrit for that I have translated all the information to English.

This Book cover information regarding treating, controlling and killing Diabetes from body, and natural method to eliminate diabetes and repairing pancreases to naturally produce insulin to control blood sugar and bring it to normal safe limit forever.

What Is Diabetes

Diabetes, often referred to by doctors as diabetes mellitus, describes a group of metabolic diseases in which the person has high blood glucose (blood sugar), either because insulin production is inadequate, or because the body's cells do not respond properly to insulin, or both. Patients with high blood sugar will typically experience polyuria (frequent urination), they will become increasingly thirsty (polydipsia) and hungry (polyphagia).

In this disease in which the body doesn't produce enough or any insulin, doesn't properly use the insulin that is produced, or exhibits a combination of both. When any of these things happens, the body is unable to get sugar from the blood into the cells. That leads to high blood sugar levels.

Glucose, the form of sugar found in your blood, is one of your main energy sources. A lack of insulin or resistance to insulin causes sugar to build up in your blood. This can lead to many health problems.

Facts on diabetes

Here are some key points about diabetes .Diabetes is a long-term condition that causes high blood sugar levels.

- In 2013 it was estimated that over 382 million people throughout the world had diabetes.
- Type 1 Diabetes - the body does not produce insulin. Approximately 10% of all diabetes cases are type 1.
- Type 2 Diabetes - the body does not produce enough insulin for proper function. Approximately 90% of all cases of diabetes worldwide are of this type.
- Gestational Diabetes - this type affects females during pregnancy.
- The most common diabetes symptoms include frequent urination, intense thirst and hunger, weight gain, unusual weight loss, fatigue, cuts and bruises that do not heal, male sexual

dysfunction, numbness and tingling in hands and feet.

- If you have Type 1 and follow a healthy eating plan, do adequate exercise, and take insulin, you can lead a normal life.
- Type 2 patients need to eat healthily, be physically active, and test their blood glucose. They may also need to take oral medication, and/or insulin to control blood glucose levels.
- As the risk of cardiovascular disease is much higher for a diabetic, it is crucial that blood pressure and cholesterol levels are monitored regularly.
- As smoking might have a serious effect on cardiovascular health, diabetics should stop smoking.
- Hypoglycemia - low blood glucose - can have a bad effect on the patient. Hyperglycemia - when blood glucose is too high - can also have a bad effect on the patient.

Different types of diabetes

The three main types of diabetes are:

- Type 1 diabetes
- Type 2 diabetes
- Gestational diabetes

1) Type 1 diabetes

The body does not produce insulin. Some people may refer to this type as insulin-dependent diabetes, juvenile diabetes, or early-onset diabetes. People usually develop type 1 diabetes before their 40th year, often in early adulthood or teenage years.

Type 1 diabetes is nowhere near as common as type 2 diabetes. Approximately 10% of all diabetes cases are type 1.

Patients with type 1 diabetes will need to take insulin injections for the rest of their life. They must also ensure proper blood-glucose levels by carrying out regular blood tests and following a special diet.

2) Type 2 diabetes

The body does not produce enough insulin for proper function, or the cells in the body do not react to insulin (insulin resistance).

Approximately 90% of all cases of diabetes worldwide are type 2.

Measuring the glucose level in blood

Some people may be able to control their type 2 diabetes symptoms by losing weight, following a healthy diet, doing plenty of exercise, and monitoring their blood glucose levels. However, type 2 diabetes is typically a progressive disease - it gradually gets worse - and the patient will probably end up have to take insulin, usually in tablet form.

Overweight and obese people have a much higher risk of developing type 2 diabetes compared to those with a healthy body weight. People with a lot of visceral fat, also known as central obesity, belly fat, or abdominal obesity, are especially at risk. Being overweight/obese causes the body to release chemicals that can destabilize the body's cardiovascular and metabolic systems.

Being overweight, physically inactive and eating the wrong foods all contribute to our risk of developing type 2 diabetes. Drinking just one can of (non-diet) soda per day can raise our risk of developing type 2 diabetes by 22%, The scientists believe that the impact of sugary soft drinks on diabetes risk may be a direct one, rather than simply an influence on body weight.

The risk of developing type 2 diabetes is also greater as we get older. Experts are not completely sure why, but say that as we age we tend to put on weight and become less physically active. Those with a close relative who had/had type 2 diabetes, people of Middle Eastern, African, or South Asian descent also have a higher risk of developing the disease.

Men whose testosterone levels are low have been found to have a higher risk of developing type 2 diabetes.

3) Gestational diabetes

This type affects females during pregnancy. Some women have very high levels of glucose in their blood, and their bodies are unable to produce enough insulin to transport all of the glucose into their cells, resulting in progressively rising levels of glucose.

Diagnosis of gestational diabetes is made during pregnancy.

The majority of gestational diabetes patients can control their diabetes with exercise and diet. Between 10% to 20% of them will need to take some kind of blood-glucose-controlling medications. Undiagnosed or uncontrolled gestational diabetes can raise the risk of complications during childbirth. The baby may be bigger than he/she should be.

Scientists found that women whose diets before becoming pregnant were high in animal fat and cholesterol had a higher risk for gestational diabetes, compared to their counterparts whose diets were low in cholesterol and animal fats.

What causes diabetes?

Type 1 diabetes

Type 1 diabetes is believed to be an autoimmune condition. This means your immune system mistakenly attacks and destroys the beta cells in your pancreas that produce insulin. The damage is permanent.

What prompts the attacks isn't clear. There may be both genetic and environmental reasons. Lifestyle factors aren't thought to play a role.

Type 2 diabetes

Type 2 diabetes starts as insulin resistance. This means your body can't use insulin efficiently. That stimulates your pancreas to produce more insulin until it can no longer keep up with demand. Insulin production decreases, which leads to high blood sugar.

The exact cause of type 2 diabetes is unknown. Contributing factors may include:

- genetics
- lack of exercise
- being overweight

There may also be other health factors and environmental reasons.

Gestational diabetes

Gestational diabetes is due to insulin-blocking hormones produced during pregnancy. This type of diabetes only occurs during pregnancy.

What is prediabetes?

The vast majority of patients with type 2 diabetes initially had prediabetes. Their blood glucose levels where higher than normal, but not high enough to merit a diabetes diagnosis. The cells in the body are becoming resistant to insulin.

Studies have indicated that even at the prediabetes stage, some damage to the circulatory system and the heart may already have occurred.

What are the symptoms?

General symptoms of diabetes include:

- excessive thirst and hunger
- frequent urination
- drowsiness or fatigue
- dry, itchy skin
- blurry vision
- slow-healing wounds

Type 2 diabetes can cause dark patches in the folds of skin in your armpits and neck. Since type 2 diabetes often takes longer to diagnose, you may feel symptoms at the time of diagnosis, like pain or numbness in your feet.

Type 1 diabetes often develops more quickly and can cause symptoms like weight loss or a condition called diabetic ketoacidosis. Diabetic ketoacidosis can occur when you have very high blood sugars, but little or no insulin in your body.

Symptoms of both types of diabetes can appear at any age, but generally type 1 occurs in children and young adults. Type 2 occurs in people over the age of 45. But younger people are increasingly being diagnosed with type 2 diabetes due to sedentary lifestyles and an increase in weight.

What are the potential complications?

Complications of diabetes generally develop over time. Having poorly controlled blood sugar levels increases the risk of serious complications that can become life-threatening. Chronic complications include

- vessel disease, leading to heart attack or stroke
- eye problems, called retinopathy
- infection or skin conditions
- nerve damage, or neuropathy
- kidney damage, or nephropathy
- amputations due to neuropathy or vessel disease

Type 2 diabetes may increase the risk of developing Alzheimer's disease, especially if your blood sugar is not well controlled.

Complications in pregnancy

High blood sugar levels during pregnancy can harm mother and child, increasing the risk of:

- high blood pressure
- preeclampsia
- miscarriage or stillbirth
- birth defects

Diabetes is a metabolism disorder

Diabetes (diabetes mellitus) is classed as a metabolism disorder. Metabolism refers to the way our bodies use digested food for energy and growth. Most of what we eat is broken down into glucose. Glucose is a form of sugar in the blood - it is the principal source of fuel for our bodies.

When our food is digested, the glucose makes its way into our bloodstream. Our cells use the glucose for energy and growth. However, glucose cannot enter our cells without insulin being present - insulin makes it possible for our cells to take in the glucose.

Insulin is a hormone that is produced by the pancreas. After eating, the pancreas automatically releases an adequate quantity of insulin to move the glucose present in our blood into the cells, as soon as glucose enters the cells blood-glucose levels drop.

A person with diabetes has a condition in which the quantity of glucose in the blood is too elevated (hyperglycemia). This is because the body either does not produce enough insulin, produces no insulin, or has cells that do not respond properly to the insulin the pancreas produces. This results in too much glucose building up in the blood. This excess blood glucose eventually passes out of the body in urine. So, even though the blood has plenty of glucose, the cells are not getting it for their essential energy and growth requirements.

How to determine whether you have diabetes, prediabetes or neither

Doctors can determine whether a patient has a normal metabolism, prediabetes or diabetes in one of three different ways - there are three possible tests:

- The A1C test
  - at least 6.5% means diabetes
  - between 5.7% and 5.99% means prediabetes
  - less than 5.7% means normal
- The FPG (fasting plasma glucose) test
  - at least 126 mg/dl means diabetes
  - between 100 mg/dl and 125.99 mg/dl means prediabetes
  - less than 100 mg/dl means normal
  An abnormal reading following the FPG means the patient has impaired fasting glucose (IFG)
- The OGTT (oral glucose tolerance test)
  - at least 200 mg/dl means diabetes
  - between 140 and 199.9 mg/dl means prediabetes
  - less than 140 mg/dl means normal

Why is it called diabetes mellitus?

Diabetes comes from Greek, and it means a "siphon". Aretus the Cappadocian, a Greek physician during the second century A.D., named the condition *diabainein*. He described patients who were passing too much water (polyuria) - like a siphon. The word became "diabetes" from the English adoption of the Medieval Latin diabetes.

In 1675, Thomas Willis added mellitus to the term, although it is commonly referred to simply as diabetes. *Mel* in Latin means "honey"; the urine and blood of people with diabetes has excess glucose, and glucose is sweet like honey. Diabetes mellitus could literally mean "siphoning off sweet water".

In ancient China people observed that ants would be attracted to some people's urine, because it was sweet. The term "Sweet Urine Disease" was coined.

Complications linked to badly controlled diabetes:

Below is a list of possible complications that can be caused by badly controlled diabetes:

- Eye complications - glaucoma, cataracts, diabetic retinopathy, and some others.
- Foot complications - neuropathy, ulcers, and sometimes gangrene which may require that the foot be amputated
- Skin complications - people with diabetes are more susceptible to skin infections and skin disorders
- Heart problems - such as ischemic heart disease, when the blood supply to the heart muscle is diminished
- Hypertension - common in people with diabetes, which can raise the risk of kidney disease, eye problems, heart attack and stroke
- Mental health - uncontrolled diabetes raises the risk of suffering from depression, anxiety and some other mental disorders

- Hearing loss - diabetes patients have a higher risk of developing hearing problems
- Gum disease - there is a much higher prevalence of gum disease among diabetes patients
- Gastroparesis - the muscles of the stomach stop working properly
- Ketoacidosis - a combination of ketosis and acidosis; accumulation of ketone bodies and acidity in the blood.
- Neuropathy - diabetic neuropathy is a type of nerve damage which can lead to several different problems.
- HHNS (Hyperosmolar Hyperglycemic Nonketotic Syndrome) - blood glucose levels shoot up too high, and there are no ketones present in the blood or urine. It is an emergency condition.
- Nephropathy - uncontrolled blood pressure can lead to kidney disease
- PAD (peripheral arterial disease) - symptoms may include pain in the leg, tingling and sometimes problems walking properly
- Stroke - if blood pressure, cholesterol levels, and blood glucose levels are not

controlled, the risk of stroke increases significantly
- Erectile dysfunction - male impotence.
- Infections - people with badly controlled diabetes are much more susceptible to infections
- Healing of wounds - cuts and lesions take much longer to heal.

Herbs for Diabetes

Shilajit

It is a thick, sticky tar-like substance with a colour ranging from white to dark brown (the latter is more common), found predominantly in Himalaya, Karakuram, Tibet mountains, Caucasus mountains, Altai Mountains, and mountains of Gilgit Baltistan .Shilajit is a blackish-brown exudation, of variable consistency, obtained from steep rocks of different formations found in the Altai MountainsIt is used in Ayurveda, the traditional Indian system of medicine. It has been reported to contain at least 85 minerals in ionic form, as well as triterpenes, humic acids and fulvic acid

Health Benefits of Shilajit

According to Ayurveda, It shield body against diabetes physical damage. Due to diabetes the body parts are damaged, it compensates for damage so that diabetic could not harm the body.

Shilajit finds extensive use in Ayurveda, for diverse clinical conditions. For centuries people living in the isolated villages in Himalaya and adjoining regions have used shilajit alone or in combination with other plant remedies to prevent and combat problems with diabetes.

Shilajit is comprised of over 85 ionic minerals and other powerful substances. One of these components is fulvic acid. Fulvic acid is beneficial in many ways, but one the most amazing effects is its ability to eradicate free-radicals. As a powerful antioxidant, it fights the oxidation of the body. It has been shown to eradicate damage to the pancreatic islet B cells done by free radicals. This damage is the leading cause for diabetes. Because the pancreas is damaged, it is unable to secrete insulin, and also isn't able to filter the toxins out of urine as effectively. Shilajit works to repair damage to the pancreas, which is then able to better release insulin and filter toxins from the body. While shilajit doesn't heal the pancreas, it provides an excellent way for diabetes patients to regulate their blood sugar levels. And, because more insulin can be released by the pancreas, glucose metabolism is encouraged.

Chemical composition

Shilajit is a herbo-mineral drug, which oozes out from a special type of mountain rocks in the peak summer months. It is found at high altitudes ranging from 1000 to 5000 meters. The active constituent of shilajit consists of dibenzo-alpha-pyrones and related metabolites, small peptides (constituting non-protein amino acids), some lipids and carrier molecules (fulvic acids). Standard shilajit contains at least 5-7% dibenzo-alpha-pyrones.

Scientific Evidence It works for Diabetes

A trial was done to study the effect of shilajit in combination with usual drugs used by diabetic patients on lipid profiles and blood glucose of diabetic rats ("Effect of shilajit on blood glucose and lipid profile in alloxan-induced diabetic rats. The result of the study, shilajit does "produced a significant reduction in blood glucose levels and also produced beneficial effects on the lipid profile." The conclusion of the study is as follows: "Shilajit is effective in controlling blood glucose levels and improves the lipid profile."

Side Effects

As you can see, shilajit has been proven to control blood sugar levels of diabetes patients. In fact, people in Nepal have been using shilajit for thousands of years to treat diabetes with great success. If you are considering using shilajit to treat and soothe the symptoms of diabetes, we advise you to consult with your doctor before doing so. Because shilajit is so effective at controlling blood sugar levels, your medicine may need to be adjusted. Additionally, urination may become more frequent after beginning the usage of shilajit – this is perfectly normal, but should be discussed with your physician before trying (there are limited shilajit side effects. If you have any questions about the benefits of shilajit for diabetes patients, don't hesitate to contact your physician to discuss how it can be used to treat and soothe your symptoms!

Gurmar (Gymnema sylvestre)

It is also called Meshshringi. Gymnema is a woody climbing shrub native to India and Africa. The leaves are used to make medicine.

Health Benefits of gurmar (Gymnema sylvestre)

It works well in diabetes. It is stimulating agent for the liver and gastric glands. This stimulates the pancreatic glands and increases the amount of insulin. It corrects the acidity of the blood due to the urine. Gymnema has a long history of use in India's Ayurvedic medicine. The Hindi name for gymnema means "destroyer of sugar." People use gymnema for diabetes, weight loss, and other conditions.

Ayurveda texts and modern research back the following facts:

- Popularly known as 'Gudmar or Gurmar' in Hindi which means 'sugar destroyer'.
- Similar to sugar molecules, the gymnemic acid in Meshashringi fills the receptor location in the absorptive layers of the intestine, interfering with sugar absorption from the intestine.
- Helps in reducing sugar levels by promoting the secretion of insulin, regenerating pancreatic cells, and increasing the activities of enzymes responsible for healthy glucose utilization.
- Provides support in achieving healthy body weight, and helps prevent triglyceride accumulation in the muscles and liver.
- Helps prevent fatty acid accumulation in the circulatory system and the hardening of blood vessels.
- Diabetes can be controlled by Gymnema Sylvestre (Meshashringi) supplement
- Diabetes is one of the slow killer disorder becoming more prevalent global. Diabetes is known for an

elevated blood sugar level due to insufficient levels of Insulin. Insulin level may be low and sugar level may be high because of many factors and till date no single medication is available to cure diabetes. Medicines control blood sugar level to normal level. Gymnema Sylvestre [Meshashringi] is one of the natural remedy from them which successfully keep sugar level to normal level.

- Meshashringi is a pure herbal extract of Gymnema Sylvestre. Also known as gurmar or periploca of the woods. Gymnema Sylvestre [Meshashringi] is popular remedy known for anti-diabetic properties. It helps to lower excessive blood sugar. Regenerative effect on pancreatic beta cells and insulinotropic activity of Meshashringi makes it more powerful anti-diabetic remedy. Regenerative effect means it stimulates the production and activity of insulin.
- Gymnema Sylvestre (Meshashringi) helps to decrease the craving for sugar. Fresh leaves have ability to numb the taste buds to the sense of sweet or bitter,

this temporarily abolishes the taste of sugar which helps to lower sugar level. Because of this sugar-destroying property, it is widely known as a "sugar destroyer".

- This all activities are due to presence of a key component of this plant Gymnema acid. Still lot of research is going on to prove effectiveness of this remedy.
- Benefits of Gymnema Sylvestre [Meshashringi]:
- Gymnema Sylvestre [Meshashringi] has been used since ancient times for multiple health benefits. These are as follows
- - Lower LDL (bad) cholesterol.
- - Improve digestion, resolve constipations.
- - Cut appetite
- - Allergies,
- - Urinary tract infections,
- - Anemia, hyperactivity,
- - Weight control.
- - Enhances the functioning of the liver.

Chemical composition

Gymnema contains substances that decrease the absorption of sugar from the intestine. Gymnema may also increase the amount of insulin in the body and increase the growth of cells in the pancreas, which is the place in the body where insulin is made.

Scientific Evidence It works for Diabetes

Early research shows that taking gymnema by mouth along with insulin or diabetes medications can improve blood sugar control in people with type 1 or type 2 diabetes.

Gymnema Sylvestre [Meshashringi] is used to treat both type of diabetes e.g. Type 1 and type 2 diabetes. It helps to maintain blood sugar level to normal level as well as normal cholesterol level. It also has no any side effects hence safe to use for long term which is beneficial to a diabetes patient. Because of this all properties Gymnema Sylvestre [Meshashringi] is getting more and more popular.

Side Effects

There are possibly no side effects with taking gurmar in small quantity.

Fenugreek seeds

Fenugreek is a plant that grows in parts of Europe and western Asia. The leaves are edible, but the small brown seeds are famous for their use in medicine. The first recorded use of fenugreek was in Egypt, dating back to 1500 B.C. Across the Middle East and South Asia, the seeds were traditionally used as both a spice and a medicine.

Health Benefits

Fenugreek is an excellent source of high soluble fibre .The seeds contain fiber and other chemicals that may slow digestion and the body's absorption of carbohydrates and sugar. The seeds may also help improve how the body uses sugar and increases the amount of insulin released. It improves glucose tolerance and also lowers blood glucose levels. Including fenugreek seeds in your daily diet may reduce the absorption of fat and cholesterol, thus providing additional cover against heart diseases and obesity. Several clinical trials have proved that fenugreek seeds can show significant improvements in the metabolic symptoms of both type 1 and type 2 diabetes.

Scientific Evidence It works for Diabetes

One study found that a daily dose of 10 grams of fenugreek seeds soaked in hot water may help control type 2 diabetes. Another study suggests that eating baked goods, such as bread, made with fenugreek flour may reduce insulin resistance in people with type 2 diabetes.

An additional study showed that taking high doses of fenugreek every day for several weeks causes noticeable improvements in plasma glucose levels. But long-term plasma glucose levels weren't measured in this study.

Side Effects

Fenugreek may also have effects on sciatic nerve issues and peripheral neuropathy. This can cause you to lose feeling in your nerves or cause your muscles to feel weak.

Some people report a maple syrup-like smell coming from their armpits after extended use. One study verified these claims by finding that certain chemicals in fenugreek, such as dimethylpyrazine, caused this smell. This smell shouldn't be confused with the smell caused by maple syrup urine disease (MUSD). This condition produces a smell that contains the same chemicals as the smells of fenugreek and maple syrup.

Fenugreek can also cause allergic reactions. Talk to your doctor about any food allergies you might have before adding fenugreek to your diet. The fiber in fenugreek can also make your body less effective at absorbing medications taken by mouth. Don't use fenugreek within a few hours of taking these types of medication. The amounts of fenugreek used in cooking are generally considered safe. When taken in large doses, side effects can include gas and bloating.

Fenugreek can also react with several medications, especially with those that treat blood clotting disorders. Talk to your doctor before taking fenugreek if you're on these types of medication

Pregnant women should limit fenugreek use to only amounts used in cooking because of its potential to induce labor.

Bimbi (Coccinia indica)

A medicine called Bimbi Coccinia indica also benefits in diabetes. Coccinia Indica also known as Bimbi in Sanskrit is a plant native to Asia, India and Central Africa. The juice of the leaves or the root are given, whose quantity is 10-20 milliliter. Bimbi that grows in the wild in most parts of India is a plant of considerable therapeutic and medicinal value. It is sometimes also called baby watermelon for its close resemblance to watermelons. Bimbi has been used for centuries in traditional Ayurveda for the treatment of diabetes, respiratory illnesses, fever, anemia, wounds, ulcers, inflammation and various skin ailments.

Health Benefits of Bimbi

Bimbi has the effect of lowering blood glucose levels in the body. Such is the potency of this herb that its performance has been compared to the standard diabetic drugs available in the market. For lowering the blood sugar, different parts of the plant are used such as the root, leaves, stem and fruit. Bimbi also controls the frequency of urination. . The extracts of the plant are known to possess antidiabetic, hypolipidemic, liver protective, antioxidant, anti-inflammatory, antitussive and antibacterial properties. The stems are used for the treatment of diabetes, UTI, bronchitis and asthma. The roots are useful in the treatment of mouth ulcers, joint pains, skin diseases and wheezing. The fruits are known to cure eczema and sores on tongue.

Chemical composition

The plant contains alkaloids, flavonoids, sterols, saponins, phytonutrients like tritriacontane, b-sitosterol, cephalandrol, lupeol, cephalandrine A, cephalandrine B and terpoenoids. The entire plant comprising of the leaves, roots and fruits are of medicinal value

Scientific Evidence It works for Diabetes

This study aimed to evaluate the effectiveness of Coccinia cordifolia on blood glucose levels of incident type 2 diabetic patients requiring only dietary or lifestyle modifications. The study was a double-blind, placebo-controlled, randomized trial. Sixty incident type 2 diabetic subjects (aged 35–60 years) were recruited. The subjects were randomly assigned into the placebo or experimental group and were provided with 1 g alcoholic extract of the herb for 90 days. Anthropometric, biochemical, dietary, and physical activity assessment were carried out at baseline and were repeated at days 45 and 90 of the study. All subjects were provided with standard dietary and physical activity advice for blood sugar control.

There was a significant decrease in the fasting, postprandial blood glucose and A1C of the experimental group compared with that of the placebo group. The fasting and postprandial blood glucose levels of the experimental group at day 90 significantly decreased, by 16 and 18%, respectively. There were no significant changes observed in the serum lipid levels.

This study suggests that Coccinia cordifolia extract has a potential hypoglycemic action in patients with mild diabetes. However, further studies are needed to elucidate mechanisms of action.

Side Effects
Bimbi is safe for most people when taken by mouth.

Haritaki (Terminalia Chebula)

Haritaki is an ayurvedic herb derived from the seeds of Terminalia Chebula tree. It is a drupe-like fruit, oval in shape with size varying between 2 – 4.5 cm in length and 1.2 – 2.5 cm in breadth having 5 longitudinal ridges. Depending upon its variety, it turns green – blackish in color when ripens. Haritaki fruit tastes sweet, sour, bitter depending upon its types. There are 7 types of Haritaki: Vijaya, Rohini, Putane, Amruta, Abhaya, Jivanti, Chetak.

Health Benefits

Haritaki has been used for centuries to reduce the fluctuations in blood glucose. Recently research has indicated that there is very strong effects using Haritaki to increase glucose tolerance and thus affect diabetes. Haritaki has been found to help Diabetes. Haritaki consists of ingredients which are recognized to have healing properties including anticancer, antibacterial, antidiabetic and anti-oxidant properties. Haritaki is also known as 'the king of medicines' and serves remarkable health benefits such as; it prevents hair loss and removes dandruff, helpful in constipation, prevent a cough and cold, removes acnes and ulcers, boost immunity, prevent diabetes, helps in weight loss, fight with skin allergies, improves heart conditions.

Chemical composition

Haritaki is very nutritious containing essential vitamins, minerals, and proteins. It is a source of vitamin C, manganese, selenium, potassium, iron and copper. It also contains plant chemicals like – tannic acid, gallic acid, palmitic acid, stearic acid and behenic acid.

Scientific Evidence It works for Diabetes

Water extract of dry fruits of Terminalia chebula at a dose of 200 mg/kg body weight improved the glucose tolerance as indicated by 44% of reduction in the peak blood glucose at 2nd hour in glucose tolerance test in diabetic (streptozotocin induced) rats.

Side Effects

The side effects of Haritaki are as follows; elimination of large amounts of built – stool, it leads to system weakening if taken with alcohol, Haritaki is not recommended if one has excessive sexual activity. Not recommended during pregnancy as its use may reduce production of breast milk.

Belpatra (Aegle marmelos)

Aegle marmelos, commonly know as bael, also Bengal quince, golden apple, japanese bitter orange, stone apple or wood apple, is a species of tree native to the Indian subcontinent and Southeast Asia. It is present in Sri Lanka, Thailand and Malesia as a naturalized species. The tree is considerd to be sacred by Hindus.

Health Benefits

Bael leaves, bel patri, bilva leaves or wood apple leaves have several medicinal benefits, controlling diabetes being just one of them. These leaves are commonly used while performing religious rituals for God Shankar or Mahadev in India. Ayurveda recognizes these as one among the dashmoola (10 herbal roots with healing properties) herb. Bael is also effective during fevers, constipation and eye infections due to its properties.

Chemical Composition

The bael tree contains furocoumarins, including xanthotoxol and the methyl ester of alloimperatorin, as well as flavonoids, rutin and marmesin; a number of essential oils

Scientific Evidence It works for Diabetes

Bael leaves are scientifically proven to have anti-diabetic properties. Bael leaf extract can reduce blood sugar and cholesterol levels along with urea. The leaf extracts also have hypoglycemic and antioxidant properties. Foods or herbs that have a low glycemic index (hypoglycemic) are known to be effective in the treatment of diabetes. The leaves also help in energizing the pancreas thus boosting the insulin production, which helps in controlling blood sugar levels.

Side Effects

There are possibly no side effects with taking Bael juice.

Bitter Gourd

It is the edible part of the plant Momordica Charantia, which is a vine of the Cucurbitaceae family and is considered the most bitter among all fruits and vegetables. The plant thrives in tropical and subtropical regions, including:

- South America
- Asia
- parts of Africa
- the Caribbean

The bitter melon itself grows off the vine as a green, oblong-shaped fruit with a distinct warty exterior - though its size, texture and bitterness vary between the different regions in which it grows - and is rich in vital vitamins and minerals

Health Benefits

Regular consumption of Bitter Gourd juice significantly improves glucose tolerance without giving any spike to insulin levels.

It makes good gains in diabetes. Its plant contains glucose, a resin and aromatic oil. It works best in diabetes. It reduces blood glucose. The action of the liver and stomach improves and stimulates the inflammation of the pancreas and increases the discharge of the insulin. By taking 10-20 ml of bitter gourd juice, it is beneficial and feeding of rice and clarified butter should be used when there is a problem of bitter gourd.

Bitter Gourd juice is an excellent beverage for diabetics. Bitter gourd helps regulate the blood sugar level in your body. Nutritionist explains, " Bitter Gourd juice makes your insulin active. When your insulin is active, your sugar would be used adequately and not convert into fat, which would eventually help in weight loss too"

Chemical composition

Bitter gourd is rich in hypoglycemic compound, which lowers sugar levels in blood. Its fruit contains ascorbic acid. In its fruits and leaves, there is a base called mocordicin. According to studies, bitter gourd has a few active substances with anti-diabetic properties. One of them is charantin, which is famous for its blood glucose-lowering effect. Bitter gourd contains an insulin-like compound called Polypeptide-p or p-insulin which has been shown to control diabetes naturally. These substances either work individually or together to help reduce blood sugar levels.

Scientific Evidence It works for Diabetes

A number of scientific studies have been conducted to evaluate the efficiency of bitter melon in the treatment of diabetes

Side effects

Use bitter gourd with caution beyond occasional use in your diet. Bitter melon can cause side effects and interfere with other medications.

Some of the risks and complications of bitter melon include:

- Diarrhea, vomiting, and other intestinal issues
- Vaginal bleeding, contractions, and abortion
- Dangerous lowering of blood sugar if taken with insulin
- Liver damage
- Favism (which can cause anemia) in those with G6PD deficiency
- Mixing with other drugs to alter their effectiveness
- Problems in blood sugar control in those who have had recent surgery

Vijayasara (Pterocarpus marsupium)

Pterocarpus marsupium, also known as Malabar kino, Indian kino tree or Vijayasar, is a medium to large, deciduous tree that can grow up to 30 metres (98 ft) tall. It is native to India, Nepal, and Sri Lanka, where it occurs in parts of the Western Ghats in the Karnataka-Keralaregion and also in the forests of Central India. It is also known by the names benga, bijiayasal (in western Nepal), piasal (Oriya), venkai, and many others

Keeping the wood of Vijayasara (Pterocarpus marsupium) in the pot, keeping the water in the night, drinking empty stomach in the morning brings relief to diabetes patients.

Health Benefits

The use of pterocarpus in the Ayurveda system of traditional medicine is thousands of years old. The aerial seeds are the most commonly used parts of the tree, including the wood, flowers and leaves. Practitioners of the Ayurveda system often use a cup made from the heartwood of pterocarpus. They fill the cup with water and allow it to stand overnight. Volatile oils in the wood leach into the water, turning it blue. This water is then drunk the next day.

The conditions commonly treated by pterocarpus in the Ayurveda system include diabetes, inflammation and bleeding. The bark is also used for bleeding and toothaches. The leaves are often applied externally as a remedy for skin diseases.

The most common uses of pterocarpus in modern herbal medicine include to help support the body's natural ability to manage and regulate blood sugar levels. Pterostilbene is one the most active ingredients of pterocarpus extract for this purpose, and other significant components include epicatechin, marsupin and pterosupin. Laboratory studies show that the gum resin of pterocarpus can help regenerate the beta cells in the pancreas.

Chemical composition

Pterostilbene, epicatechin, pterosupin, marsupsin, etc., have been identified and isolated. Pterocarpus marsupium extract shows promising results in cataract and hypertriglyceridaemia. This plant has various pharmacological activities like anti-diabetic, antifungal, antioxidant, analgesic, anti-inflammatory, hepatoprotective etc.

Scientific Evidence It works for Diabetes

A scientific study was designed to investigate the effect of aqueous extract of *Pterocarpus marsupium* on elevated inflammatory cytokine, tumor necrosis factor (TNF)-α in type 2 diabetic rats

The result of study was that Aqueous extract of *P. marsupium* at both doses, i.e., 100 and 200 mg/kg, decreased the fasting and postprandial blood glucose in type 2 diabetic rats.

Side Effects

There are no side effects with taking Vijayasara.

Giloy (Tinospora Cordifolia/ Guduchi/ Amrita Satva)

"Giloy (Tinospora Cordifolia) is an Ayurvedic herb that has been used and advocated in Indian medicine for ages. In

Sanskrit, Giloy is known as 'Amrita', which literally translates to 'the root of immortality', because of its abundant medicinal properties. "The stem of Giloy is of maximum utility, but the root can also be used "Giloy can be consumed in the form of juice, powder or capsules".

Giloy acts as a hypoglycaemic agent and helps treat diabetes (particularly Type 2 diabetes)". Giloy juice helps reduce high levels of blood sugar and works wonders

Health Benefits

- Giloy is a good remedy to boost immunity. It has antioxidants which fight damaging free radicals. Diabetic patients are vulnerable to immunological deficiency.
- The herb helps acts as an immunomodulator to control glycemia in the body.
- It is a natural anti-diabetic medicine. It acts as a hypoglycaemic agent for diabetes mellitus patients.

- High blood pressure and lipid can easily control through this herb.
- Intake of Guduchi will help suppress craving for sugar.
- The herb helps in the production of beta cells of the pancreas. They result in smooth regulation of insulin and glucose in the blood.
- The anti-inflammatory and anti-arthritic properties are helpful in the diabetic condition of joint pain, swelling, arthritis. It is helpful in cases of diabetic neuropathic arthropathy or diabetic osteoarthropathy.
- Eye related problems can be prevented and cured to some extents using Giloy.
- Giloy has been found beneficial for the digestive system. It improves laxation in the body. The bowel movement is improved.
- As per a report, people have said that they feel light after taking giloy. It is due to their adaptogenic properties. It helps relieve stress, anxiety, and depression.

Chemical composition

It is abundant in alkaloids. Diterpenes are of great interest for their number and chemistry. The other bio-chemical substances, which are found in giloy are steroids, flavonoids, lignans, carbohydrates, etc. Its bio-chemical products are used in the manufacturing of many herbal, ayurvedic and modern medicines.

Scientific Evidence It works for Diabetes

Scientific Research shows that Giloy gives immediate and beneficial effect in glucose tolerance and adrenaline induced Hyperglycaemia. It helps in the production of insulin and enhances the capacity to burn glucose. It decreases the blood sugar level.

Side Effects

Consuming too much giloy causes constipation and stomach irritation. These side effects will occur irrespective of what form of giloy you consume - juice or supplement capsule.

Banyan tree (Ficus Bengalensis)

Ficus benghalensis, commonly known as the banyan, banyan fig and Indian banyan, is a tree native to the Indian Subcontinent. Specimens in India are among the largest trees in the world by canopy coverage. Ficus benghalensis produces propagating roots which grow downwards as aerial roots. Once these roots reach the ground they grow into woody trunks.

The figs produced by the tree are eaten by birds such as the Indian myna. Fig seeds that pass through the digestive system of birds are more likely to germinate and sprout earlier.

Health Benefits

Banyan tree which is also known as Ficus Bengalensis has very effective Body sugar level reducing property. By eating its bark regularly, you can make your diabetes disappear. This is a very simple method. This is the traditional but very effective way to knock out sugar levels in your body. These methods are practiced during over good olden days when there are no such medicines and insulin which we are taking now.This remedy can surely knock out your diabetes if you practice regularly keeping faith on it.

Chemical composition

The fruits of ficus Bengalensis contain water (92%), carbohydrates (4-6%), protein (1-2%), minerals (1%) and a moderate amount of vitamins, mainly A and C

Scientific Evidence It works for Diabetes

A number of scientific studies have been conducted to evaluate the efficiency of Banyan tree bark in the treatment of diabetes

Side Effects

There are no side effects with taking Banyan tree bark or aerial roots.

Turmeric

Turmeric is a spice made from the ground roots of the turmeric plant. Over the years, turmeric has been recognized for its medicinal properties. It's believed to have a wide range of health benefits, including pain relief and possible disease prevention.

For example, curcumin, the active component in turmeric, may help prevent type 2 diabetes.

Health Benefits

Turmeric is a spice often found in Asian food and curries. It helps give the food its yellowish color. For centuries, it has been used in Eastern medicine for general health. It's often used for improving liver and digestion functions, as well as for easing pain from conditions such as arthritis.

The spice has a large following among alternative medicine users and is gaining popularity in mainstream medicine. Recently, it has received a lot of attention for its potential use in preventing cancer and other diseases. Turmeric is believed to have antioxidant properties that could help fight infection and inflammation.

Research has also suggested that taking turmeric could treat and prevent diabetes.

Chemical composition

Turmeric include a 26% daily value in manganese and 16% in iron. It's also an excellent source of fiber, vitamin B6, potassium, and healthy amounts of vitamin C and magnesium.

Scientific Evidence It works for Diabetes

Turmeric's active component, curcumin, is credited with many of the spice's purported benefits. 2013 studies suggests that curcumin can decrease the level of glucose in blood, as well as other diabetes-related complications. Researchers also found that curcumin may have a role in diabetes prevention. More clinical trials with humans are needed for a better understanding of curcumin and turmeric's effects. Other research suggests that turmeric extract could help stabilize blood sugar levels and make diabetes more manageable. This extract can be found in over-the-counter supplements. It may also provide general health benefits, such as in aiding digestion.

Side Effects

Repeatedly consuming large amounts of turmeric may cause liver problems. If you have gallbladder disease, you should avoid turmeric. It may worsen your condition. Consult with your doctor before using turmeric. They can assess your medical profile and discuss the potential benefits and risks.

Turmeric is generally regarded as safe for consumption. When curcumin, the active component of turmeric, is taken in large doses — more than is typically consumed in a meal flavored with turmeric — it may cause unpleasant side effects. A high dosage is typically considered above 4 grams of curcumin daily.

Arjun tree bark (Terminalia arjuna)

"Terminalia arjuna."z is a Ayurvedic herb has been used medicinally for thousands of years. In a recent clinical trial, researchers in India discovered that arjuna demonstrates "remarkable hyperglycemic activity."

Health Benefits

It is one of the most important heart herbs in Ayurvedic medicine. Arjuna is thought to reduce heart-damaging inflammation and mucous. It has been used to treat angina pectoris, hypercholesterolemia, cardiac artery disease, and hypertension.

Chemical composition

The bark extract contains acids (arjunic acid, terminic acid), glycosides (arjunetin arjunosides I-IV), antioxidants (flavones, tannins, oligomeric, proanthocyanidins), and minerals.

Scientific Evidence It works for Diabetes

This health news comes via an animal study. The researchers set out to evaluate the anti-hyperglycemic and antioxidant role of arjuna leaf extract in rats. After hyperglycemia was induced in the rats, they were given either the arjuna extract or "Glibenclamide," a popular anti-diabetic drug.

The researchers found that arjuna extract reduced and normalized blood glucose levels much more effectively compared to Glibenclamide. They also noted that arjuna extract significantly decreased cell damage caused by free radicals. They concluded that arjuna leaf demonstrated remarkable anti-hyperglycemic activity. The researchers speculated that the anti-hyperglycemic action is likely due to arjuna's antioxidant content.

Side Effects

Terminalia arjuna is safe when taken by mouth.

Neem

Neem is a tropical plant that grows extensively across India. Neem trees are nearly 30-50 feet high, and almost every part of the tree is profuse with antiseptic and healing properties. Neem has been an integral part of Indian and Chinese medicine since time immemorial.

Health Benefits

Almost all parts of the neem tree- leaves, flowers, seeds, fruits, roots and bark have been used traditionally for a variety of treatments; be it inflammation, infections, fever, skin diseases or dental disorders. Some studies have claimed that certain compounds of Azadirachta indica (Neem) could be of benefit in diabetes mellitus in controlling the blood sugar. According to a study, neem may also prove helpful in preventing or delaying the onset of the disease. Neem leaf powder was found to control diabetic symptoms on non-insulin dependent male diabetics too.

If you have diabetes, you can have neem juice daily, or just chew into a handful of neem leaves. Make sure you do not overdo it neem leaves have hypoglycaemic effect.

Chemical composition

Neem leaves are loaded with flavonoids, triterpenoid, anti-viral compounds and glycosides, which may help manage blood sugar levels and ensure there is no surge in glucose.

Scientific Evidence It works for Diabetes

According to studies, Neem plant has hypoglycaemic or blood sugar lowering properties. Therefore, Neem is beneficial in controlling the blood sugar levels and can be ideal for diabetic patients. It can also delay and prevent certain diseases. It also prevents oxidative stress which is caused due to diabetes. Anti-diabetic properties in neem oil or neem extracts make it useful for maintaining a healthy body.

Side Effects

Neem shouldn't be consumed by infants because it contains certain substances which is known to cause Reye's syndrome in infants. Even a small dosage can prove fatal for them. It can also cause allergies, infertility, miscarriages in women and stomach irritation. It can also cause kidney damage if it is taken excessively and can increase fatigue. People with already low blood pressure are advised not to consume Neem.

Kalmegha (Green chiretta or Andrographis paniculata)

Kalmegha commonly know as green chiretta or Andrographis paniculata is an annual herbaceous plant in the family Acanthaceae, native to India and Sri Lanka.

It is widely cultivated in Southern and Southeastern Asia, where it has been traditionally used to treat infections and some diseases. Mostly the leaves and roots were used for medicinal purposes. The whole plant is also used in some cases

Health Benefits

Kalmegha is basically a forest herb known for its bitterness which can control Diabetes effectively which is also very effective for diseases like Malaria, Dengue, liver problems, digestive disorders and all types of skin diseases because Kalmegha mainly works with blood purification system. Due to Kalmegha's bitter taste there is a jovial say that 'neither animal eat it nor thieves take it'.

If one become immune to its consumption about two table spoon everyday they are free from problems like common cold, cough, fever, bodyache, skin diseases it is also heard that it is good for vitiligo.

Chemical composition

The plant contains andrographolide, neoand, andrographolide, deoxy-andrographolide, andrographiside. The leaves contain active principle like andrographolide, homo-andrographolide andrographesterol and andrographone. Andrographolide is is the major constituent in leaves which is bitter substance.

Scientific Evidence It works for Diabetes

A number of scientific studies have been conducted to evaluate the efficiency of kalmegha in the treatment of diabetes

Side Effects

There are no side effects with taking kalmegha

Kali jeeri (Black Cumin Seeds)

Kali Jeeri -- also known as kalijiri, bitter cumin or Centratherum anthelminticum -- is a plant, and its seeds are sometimes used as an herbal medicine. It shouldn't be confused with two other types of cumin Bunium persicum, also called kala jeera, and Nigella sativa both sometimes referred to as black cumin. Black cumin seeds are different from normal cumin seeds. It is known as kala jeera in India and the scientific name is Nigella sativa.

Health Benefits

1. Black cumin seeds are effective in the treatment of diabetes.
2. It is used for the treatment of epilepsy and other disorders related to the nervous system.
3. Black cumin seeds are used to treat respiratory disorders such as bronchitis and asthma.
4. Studies prove that the black cumin seeds are effective in prevention of colon cancer

or cancer in the digestive system.
5. Black cumin seeds help to regulate menstruation.
6. Black cumin seeds help to maintain healthy skin.
7. It has antibiotic property, thus can use in case of bacterial infections.
8. Black cumin seeds help in maintaining blood pressure and it provides protection to the heart.
9. It is effective in the prevention of cancer such as breast cancer, oral cancer, leukemia and brain tumour.
10. It can be used in the case of diarrhoea and constipation.
11. Black cumin seeds are useful in the nursing mother to stimulate breast milk.

Chemical composition

Black cumin contains 20.85% protein, 38.20% fat, 4.64% moisture, 4.37% ash, 7.94% crude fibre and 31.94% total carbohydrates. Potassium, phosphorus, sodium and iron were the predominant elements present in it.

Scientific Evidence It works for Diabetes

An animal study found that kali jeeri may have the ability to increase insulin secretion and thus lower high blood sugar levels in diabetics. Another study found that finding kali jeeri is capable of lowering blood sugar levels with potentially fewer side effects than the diabetes medication Glibenclamide.

Side effects

Kaali jeeri when taken in overdose can cause a number of side effects, including diarrhoea, vomiting, stomach cramps, joint pain, dizziness, rash and weakness. High doses of it can make you dehydrated and cause an electrolyte imbalance that can give you an irregular heartbeat. Certain people, including those with diabetes, kidney problems, pancreatitis or gout, should avoid using it, as they could make these conditions worse.

Amla (Phyllanthus emblica)

Phyllanthus emblica, also known as emblic, emblic myrobalan, myrobalan, Indian gooseberry, Malacca tree, or amla from Sanskrit amalaki is a deciduous tree of the family Phyllanthaceae. It is known for its edible fruit of the same name.

Health Benefits

1. Slows Down Ageing
2. Cures A Sore Throat
3. Fights Against Heart Disease
4. Increases Diuretic Activity
5. Increases Metabolic Activity
6. Reduces Blood Sugar
7. High In Digestive Fiber
8. Boosts Immunity
9. Prevents Formation Of Gall Bladder Stones
10. Prevents Ulcers

11. Is Anti-Inflammatory

12. Improves Eyesight

13. Purifies Blood

14. Strengthens Bones

15. Cools The Body

16. Prevents Constipation

17. Prevents Jaundice

18. Reduces The Risk Of Cancer

19. Protects Your Liver

20. Makes Skin Glow

21. Brightens Skin

22. Reduces Pigmentation

23. Prevents Lice

24. Prevents Greying Of Hair

25. Helps Increase Hair Growth

Chemical composition

Amla contain high amounts of ascorbic
acid (vitamin C), up to 445 mg per
100 g, the specific contents are disputed, and
the overall bitterness of amla may derive
instead from its high density
of ellagitannins, such as emblicanin A
(37%), emblicanin B

(33%), punigluconin (12%)
and pedunculagin (14%). It also
contains punicafolin and phyllanemblinin A,
phyllanemblin other polyphenols, such
as flavonoids, kaempferol, ellagic acid,
and gallic acid.

Scientific Evidence It works for Diabetes
For those suffering from diabetes, Amla is a
good source of Vitamin C, which is required
for repairing of pancreatic tissues. It also
further prevents the damage of insulin
producing cells. Amla contains chromium
that regulates the carbohydrate metabolism
in your body. Consumption of amla may
make your body more responsive to Insulin.
You can have one raw amla once in a day,
but avoid processed forms of amla,
especially those that have added sugar, as
they can aggravate blood sugar levels.

Side effects

Overdosing with amla can cause increased
risk of bleeding or bruising in some people.

If you have a bleeding disorder, use Indian gooseberry with caution.

Some More herbs for diabetes

Kadamb tree (Neolamarckia cadamba)

Chiraayata (Swertia)

Indrajav (Holarrhena pubescens)

Ashwagandha (Withaniasomnifera)

Gokharu (Tribululsterrestris)

Kachur (Curcuma zedoaria)

Jamun (Syzygiumcumini)

Chirayata (Swertiachirata)

Kutki (Picrorhiza Kurroa)

Kuchla Shudh (Strychnos Nux- vomica)

Ativisha (Aconitum heterophyllum)

Indrayad (Citrullus colocynthis)

Saras (Albizia lebbeck)

Katira Gum (Tragacanth Gum)

Makhana (Prickly Water Lily or Euryale ferox)

Gudhal (hibiscus)

Aloe vera

Binaula khal (cotton seed)

Chitrak (plumbago zeylanica)

Shankahuli or shakhpushpi (Convolvulus pluricaulis choisy)

Sheetalchini or Kababchini (Piper cubeba)

Tulsi (Holy Basil)

Tejpatta (Bay Leaf)

Trivang Bhasma

Mahua Tree (Madhuca longifolia)

Betel Leaf

Amaltaash Tree (cassia)

Suva Bhaaji (Dill leaf)

Nagarmotha (Cyperus scariosus)

Lodhra (Symplocos)

Kaaya Fruit (Box myrtle or Myrica esculenta)

Jastha-Bhasma (zinc bhasma)

Pashanbhed (Coleus Forskohlii or Plectranthus barbatus)

Sadabahar Tree (Madagascar Periwinkle or Catharanthus roseus)

Triphala

Saptakriya

Natural treatment for diabetes

The real reason of diabetes is that the amount of fat (dirty cholesterol) LDL in your blood increases, then the cholesterol in the blood sticks to the cells! After which the insulin is not able to reach the cells (the amount of insulin is adequate but it cannot reach to insulin receptors of cells and after that the insulin receptors are reduced)

The insulin does not come in any work for the body, because of which when we check the sugar level, the level of sugar always stays increased in the body because it does not reach the cell because there is (dirty cholesterol) LDL VLDL accumulated. But when we take insulin out from the outside, then that insulin is new, then it reaches inside the cells!

The discussion of diabetes is happening much more nowadays, because of this secretly knocking disease, it is increasing rapidly that people are not able to understand. It does not happen after eating sugar but after that you Should not eat sugar, it is true.

And the second thing is that there is no solution to the quencher's food. It is just the conspiracy of consoling the mind, there may be something in the stomach that works on diabetes such as bitter gourd, Gurmar (Gymnema sylvestre), Swertia.

In diabetes only those herbs are effective which can revitalize the weakened cell or dead cell of the pancreas or create the power to release insulin from it. Some Medicines are also effective, such as Jamun's seeds, Vijayasar, Shelf, Tulsi leaf.

Herbs like Shilajit, Saptakriya, Bimbi, Vijaysaar Tree Bark, fenugreek seeds, Gurmar (Gymnema sylvestre), Swertia etc. are used for Treating type 1 and type 2 diabetes.

Secret To kill Diabetes Forever

All the Herbs listed above are hypoglycaemic in nature as proved by scientific evidence, but one thing they and you do not know that if you take these Herbs for a period from 1 to 3 month on regular basis will completely knock out diabetes from your life. But in that period you have to stop consuming sugar or its products completely. The Indian sages had told this already in Vedas. If you could understand Indian Vedas which in written in Vedic Sanskrit, then you will discover all the secret of this world for any field.

Most Effective Method To Remove diabetes

Kadamb Tree Leaves Recipe

Take 15 to 20 leaves of Kadamb tree (Neolamarckia cadamba), crush them or grind them to make a paste then put this paste in Tea making vessel and add 1 cup of water and boil this solution on medium flame until half cup of water is remained and filter the solution and drink it in every morning and evening one hour before and after eating food and avoid sugar and its products completely. Take this solution from 1 to 2 month daily to completely knock out diabetes. This is the most effective and fast method to knock out diabetes from all the Method.

Kalmegha Tree Leaves Recipe

Take 20 leaves of Kalmegha (Green chiretta or Andrographis paniculata), boil the leaves in one cup of water, when the water becomes half cup, remove the leaves drink the water, hardly two or three times, and you are free from Diabetes. Kalmegha is also available in powder form online.

Banyan Tree Anti-Diabetic Recipe

1. Take the bark of Banyan tree (Ficus Bengalensis).
2. Dry the bark under sunlight
3. Take powder out of it and store it in a tight container
4. Mix 1 teaspoon of this powder with 1 glass of water to make a   Decoction
5.This mixture is then simmered slowly for 15 to 20 minutes or until it becomes half cup of water
6.Filter this half cup of decoction
7.Take this Luke warm decoction daily to completely knock out your diabetes

Fenugreek seeds, Jamun seeds and Belpatra leaves Antidiabetic Recipe

Take 100 grams (Fenugreek seeds) and dry it in the sun and grind it on the stone and make powder.

Take 100 grams (Bay Leaves), dry it in the sun and grind it on the stone and make powder.

Take 150 grams (Jamun Seeds), dry it in the sun and grind it on the stone and make powder.

Take 250 grams (leaves of Beael), dry it in the sun and grind it on the stone and make powder.

Make powder of all these herbs and mix them all together. Your medicine is ready.

Take one and half teaspoon of it with hot water for one hour before eating it from morning (empty stomach).

Take it 2 to 3 months continuously (Take it after clearing the stomach in the morning) to completely knock out diabetes.

Triphala powder

Triphala means three fruits!

1) Harad (Terminalia chebula)
2) Baheda (Terminalia bellirica)
3) Amla (Emblica officinalis)

Remember one thing should always be 1: 2: 3! 1 ratio 2 ratio 3!

First of all, take 100 grams of Harad, then 200 grams of Baheda and 300 grams of Amla.
Make powder of all of them and take one and half spoon tablespoon with hot milk at night to 2 to 3 month to completely knock out diabetes.

Haritaki powder

In Every morning and evening consume 1 tea spoon of Haritaki (Terminalia chebula) powder with a little honey. Constant intake of Haritaki helps to control diabetes.

Saptakriya

Saptakriya which is called Hippocrateacei in English, the quantity of its Decoction is taken 50-100 milliliters. It is used in diabetes. This reduces urine and also reduces the amount of sugar in the blood. In addition, improves the patient's health.

Bael leaves

Chew 4-5 Bael leaves every morning on an empty stomach. Continuing this routine for a prolonged time keeps diabetes in check. Bael leaves juice can be extracted by mixing them with little water in the blender. This juice is more effective if taken with a pinch of pepper. You can also chew both Bael and Basil leaves together to help keep diabetes and cholesterol in control. Bael fruits or leaves should be avoided during pregnancy. Please consult your doctor in case you are pregnant or planning to conceive.

Green onion Recipe

Take 3 to 4 big green onion with its roots, wash them properly and put them in two litre of water for full night and drink this water in morning, don't drink this water at once, Drink this water only when you are thirsty. By following this for 1 month you will knock out diabetes.

Mango tree leaves Recipe

Take 100 to 300 grams of Fresh mango tree (Mangifera Indica) leaves, dry the in shade and grind them to make powder, take 1 tea spoon of this powder with water empty stomach or take 1 tea spoon of this powder and boil to 1 cup of water and boil till half cup water remains and filter the water and drink with empty stomach to completely knock out diabetes.

Bitter Gourd Juice Recipe

Peel the bitter gourd with the help of a knife. Slice the bitter gourd to the centre. Once you are done slicing, scoop out the white flesh and the seeds of the vegetable. Now, take the bitter gourd and cut them into tiny pieces. Soak the pieces in cold water for about 30 minutes. Add bitter gourd pieces to a juicer and add half teaspoon of salt and lemon juice. Blend the ingredients.

Add lemon juice to lessen the harsh taste of bitter gourd juice. A pinch of black pepper and ginger can also decrease the tartness and make it more palatable. Drink this juice daily to control sugar level under normal limit.

Neem Leaves juice Recipe

1. Wash about 20 neem (Azadirachta indica) leaves in half a litre of hot water for about 5 minutes.

2. You would see that the leaves have begun to appear soft. The water will gradually turn deep green in colour.

3. Take out the leaves, grind them with 1 glass of water and filter the solution and drink it with empty stomach in every morning and evening.

4. follow this method for one to two month and you can control diabetes.

Yunnan Recipe

Take 50 gram Indrayan fruit (Citrullus colocynthis), 50 gram Saras seed (Albizia lebbeck) and 50 Kateera Gum (Tragacanth Gum), make powder of all these ingredients and mix them well and take empty capsules and fill all the powder taking 1 gram quantity in each capsule and take 1 capsule in morning and evening with empty stomach for 2 month to knock out diabetes.

Black cumin and Fenugreek seeds recipe

Take 100 grams Black cumin seeds and 100 gram Fenugreek seeds and grind them and mix them together and put this mixture in a jar. At every night take one tea spoon of this mixture and put in 1 glass of water and mix it well, leave it for whole night and in morning drink this solution with empty stomach and chew the mixture well, follow this method for 2 to 3 month to knock out any level of diabetes.

Makhana Recipe

Eating 4 Makhana (Prickly Water Lily or Euryale ferox) with empty stomach in every morning will control sugar level to bring it to normal.

Hibiscus Leaves Recipe

Take 200 grams of fresh Hibiscus leaves and dry them in shade, after they are dried make fine powder of them and take 3 to 4 tea spoon of this powder and mix it with 1 glass of water and take with empty stomach in every morning for 10 to 15 days to fully control diabetes.

Sahejan Leaves Recipe

Take 100 grams Sahejan (Drumstick tree or Moringa oleifera) leaves, dry them in shade and make fine powder and take 2 to 3 tea spoon and mix with one glass of water and drink 1 hour before and after having food. This is natural insulin for diabetic people. If followed for 2 month then diabetes will be controlled.

Jamun seed and Gurmar Recipe

Take 100 grams of jamun (Java plum or Syzygium cumini) seeds and 100 grams of Gurmar (Gymnema sylvestre), grind them to make fine powder, take 1 teaspoon three times per day with Aloe vera juice and follow this method for 1 month to knock out diabetes.

Giloy and Pashanbhed

Take 40 grams of Green Giloy (Guduchi or Tinospora cordofolia) Leaves, 6 grams of Pashanbhed (Coleus Forskohlii or Plectranthus barbatus) and 6 grams of pure Honey and mix them well or make paste and take it every morning and evening before having food for 1 month to knock out diabetes.

Shilajit Recipe

Take 5 grams of pure Shilajit and drink it with one glass of milk every day to knock out diabetes. Follow this method until you have consumed minimum of one kilogram of pure shilajit. Do this procedure only in winter. This method will knock out diabetes and control it.

Binaula Khal Recipe

Take 20 gram of Binaula khal (cotton seeds) and crush it and put in 600 grams boiling water. When one fourth water remained then filter this water and take 10 grams of this water for 3 to 4 times per day to control diabetes.

Chitrak recipe

Take 6 gram Chitrak (plumbago zeylanica) powder and boil it in 500 gram of water when 300 gram of water remained then filter the water and drink it when it become luke warm. Only after 3 weeks diabetes will be knocked out completely.

Sheetalchini, Gurmar and Ashwagandha Recipe

Take 50 grams Gurmar (Gymnema sylvestre), 50 gram Sheetalchini (Piper cubeba), 50 gram Ashwandha and 50 gram shankhahuli (Convolvulus pluricaulis choisy), mix them altogether and make fine powder and take 3 gram of this powder 3 times daily with empty stomach with one glass water to knock out diabetes.

Black pepper and kaali jeeri recipe

Take Black pepper 20 grams, Kaali jeeri (Bitter cumin, Black cummin or Centratherum anthelminticum) 20 grams, Basil leaves 20 grams and rock salt 10 grams, mix them and make fine powder, take half tea spoon daily every morning and evening with one glass water. After 1 month you will knock out diabetes.

Bitter gourd and Gurmar recipe

Take one glass of Bitter gourd juice and mix with 3 to 6 grams Gurmar (Gymnema sylvestre) powder and drink it every morning and evening for one and half month to knock out diabetes.

Turmeric and Honey Recipe

Take 3 grams of Turmeric powder with 12 grams of pure Honey for 3 month to knock out diabetes.

Mahua Tree bark and Black pepper Recipe

Take 5 gram of Mahua (Madhuca longifolia) tree bark and 1 gram of black pepper, Make powder of altogether and drink with one glass of water in every morning and evening with empty stomach to knock out diabetes.

Bael leaves and Black pepper Recipe

Take 20 grams of fresh Bael leaves and 110 grams black pepper mix them and grind them and take it daily to knock out diabetes.

Bael leaves and honey Recipe

Take 250 grams Bael leaves juice and mix with honey and drink it every morning when you wake up with empty stomach to knock out diabetes.

Betel Leaf and zinc bhasma Recipe

Eating Betel leaves with Jastha-bhasma (Zinc Bhasma) will knock out diabetes.

Giloy, Honey and Pashanbhed Recipe

Take 6 grams Pashanbhed (Coleus Forskohlii or Plectranthus barbatus), 40 grams fresh of Giloy (Guduchi or Tinospora cordofolia) juice and 6 gram pure honey mix them all together and take for 1 month to completely knock out diabetes.

Babul Gum and Milk Recipe

Take 3 grams of Babul Gum (Gum Arabic tree) powder and take with 1 glass milk to control diabetes.

Indrajav Seeds Recipe

Take 100 gram of Indrajav (Holarrhena pubescens) Seeds and make fine powder of it and take 1 tea spoon or mix 2 teaspoon of indrajav in two glass of water at night and drink in every morning and evening with empty stomach to knock out diabetes in one month.

Vijaysar Tree bark Recipe

Take 20 gram of Vijaysar (Pterocarpus marsupium) tree bark and make it fine powder and boil it in 1 glass of water and filter it when half glass of water remained and drink it every morning and evening with empty stomach for 1 to 2 months to knock out diabetes.

Conclusion

Thank you for making it through to the end of "Knock out Diabetes in one month", I hope it was informative and was able to provide you with all remedies you need to get rid of Diabetes.

The next step is to start trying some of these remedies for your kidney stone disease. Start with one or two and see what works best to dissolve kidney stone fast. Make sure that you follow recommended doses, Indication and warning; otherwise, you may not get any benefit. It's also a good idea to talk to your doctor first.

Finally, if you found this Book useful in any way, a review on amazon is always appreciated!

This book is to help people eliminate Diabetes from body You can find the Herbs given in this Book online or you can buy them from herbs shop or you can find them in nature easily. For more information regarding the herbs given in this book online search can be performed to know more about any particular herb or its added benefits.

For more information check our
Facebook page:
www.facebook.com/Health.fitness.blogg
Twitter : www.twitter.com/Hbloggg
Instagram:
www.instagram.com/Health.fitness.bloggg
Website: www.healthfitnessblogg.com

www.ingramcontent.com/pod-product-compliance
Lightning Source LLC
Chambersburg PA
CBHW070026260726
48658CB00002B/505